Table of Contents

Understanding and Addressing Postpartum Depression

The Baby Blues vs. Postpartum Depression: Similarities and Differences

1. Introduction

Although many women expect that childbirth will bring great happiness, many also feel depressed and angry for days, weeks, months, or even years after delivery. The "baby blues" and clinical postpartum depression are different in their severity and duration of such emotions. These periods of sadness (the blues and clinical depression) have a profound impact on mothers and on their families. The purpose of the following information is to help you distinguish between these two conditions and to help you know when to seek assistance and what types of help are available.

You can imagine it: no sleep, the feelings of confusion, and the day to day changes that accompany becoming a new parent. Most mothers experience many of the above symptoms. During the first couple of weeks after birth, a woman's body has to quickly readjust to normal hormone fluctuations and make the transition from 2 bodies in 1 to its new state of 1 body. The purpose of a New Mother's class is to educate you about this time of transition for your body and to provide information on the support that is available to you and your family. The handout you are about to read gives you a feel for the difference between the "baby blues" and perhaps clinical postpartum depression. In addition, it describes what a mother's symptoms may mean for her family and identifies limits to a mother's ability to safely care for her children.

2. Understanding the Baby Blues

The Baby Blues can be a very confusing time for new mothers, mainly due to the fact that the people around us expect us to be happy, as we have just become a mum or added to our family. However, in reality, new mothers can experience overwhelming feelings of sadness, emotional sensitivity, guilt, ambivalence, and tension all at the same time. It is normal for a new mother to go through a grieving process as she comes to terms with having to say goodbye to her old lifestyle and say hello to life with her new baby. It is also normal to be feeling overwhelmed, tired, physically unwell, and even slightly anxious.

The Baby Blues is a term used to describe feelings of sadness, anxiety, irritability, and worry experienced by new mothers in the first two weeks postpartum. These feelings, which can range from moderate to severe, are considered to be a normal part of adjusting to life with a new baby. It is thought that about 30% to 80% of women experience the Baby Blues. Symptoms generally peak in the first four to five days and then pass within a few days to a week, and very rarely can they last for two weeks. Every time we experience an event that is emotionally or physically demanding, a hormone is released in the brain. Research has shown that women who are pregnant experience an increase of these two hormones by the end of their pregnancy. After giving birth, the levels of the hormones are much the same as the hormones released from the stressor hormone. This release of the stressor hormone after the stressor is removed could put the new mum at risk of experiencing the Baby Blues.

2.1. Definition and Characteristics

The so-called baby blues is temporary and refers to mothers who have occasional incontestable despair and crying, but it generally goes away after a few weeks. Baby blues is, therefore, characterized by a lot of crying, irritability, lack of patience, and difficulty falling asleep when from one to three days after birth up to 2-3 weeks after birth. Although associated with the emotional outburst of the mothers, the baby blues should not be confused, especially by the health personnel, with depression. The symptoms related to the baby blues are characterized by verbosity, egocentrism, and an intractable resentfulness. They are not automatically attributable to incompatibilities between the mother and baby; however, the lack of sleep may exacerbate them. During the time she undergoes the baby blues, the new mother is prey to fears: would she be a good mother to her baby? At the same time, indirectly, she is afraid that the child may realize the maternal anxieties and may suffer from the lack of attention and love.

During this subsection, we are going to describe the concept and the typical features of the baby blues. Baby Blues have an onset, for a large part of the baby blues cases, within the first 3 days after birth, and even the first 3 days to 2 weeks after birth. It is interesting to observe the individual's response to the birth of the child: it is quite variable. If a child was longed for, he may actually awaken joyful feelings in the parents, but often he also disappoints because he is not perfect or because he is not what one hoped for: there are some children who are desired as boys and instead are female and vice versa. Disappointment is also common if the child does not have certain features: for example, in the case of white families, there are mothers who are very disappointed if their child is born black.

2.2. Prevalence and Duration

Women note that in those early days and weeks after having a baby, there are days that can be better or worse for them in terms of their symptoms. However, for most women, whether they have felt really "bluesy," anxious, or irritable, they start to feel more like themselves again by the end of the third week postpartum. It is not unusual, however, if a woman feels like she is sliding into a really intense blues spell at some other time between the 3rd and the 6th week postpartum before feeling normal again.

According to a national survey of nearly 800 women, 76% of women report having symptoms of the baby blues in the first days and weeks after having a baby. Some women describe only having these symptoms for a few hours a day; others note that these symptoms last most of the day and they feel as though their moods are just "all over the place." One of the unique things about the baby blues is that they come and go. However, even when they come back, they seem to be a bit less intense.

3. Exploring Postpartum Depression

Just like the baby blues, this form of depression is nothing for a new mom to be embarrassed about. Modern medical science is beginning to understand the reason why some women experience a severe hormonal imbalance following childbirth. In addition to postpartum depression itself carrying a long list of symptoms, something like this can also lead to other mood disorders and mental health conditions caused by long-term physical issues – many of which are connected to having and recovering from childbirth. Postpartum depression can interfere with the mother's ability to connect with her baby. Instead of being able to bond with the newborn, a mom suffering from PPD may be overwhelmed by feelings of guilt, shame, or inadequacy. Bonding with the baby on an emotional level might become difficult for a suffering mother due to the mother's inability to produce feelings that are needed for making that emotional attachment. Instead of feeling proud of motherhood or simply just loving their newborn, mothers might feel resentment or dread at the thought of having to care for them.

One of the biggest telltale signs that a woman is suffering from postpartum depression and not simply the baby blues is the severity of the symptoms. Postpartum depression is a mood disorder that can make it incredibly difficult for a new mom to handle each day. This condition occurs in some women and generally begins sometime during the first six months following childbirth. Mothers who are unable to find the help they need for postpartum depression can end up struggling with the condition for months or even years after childbirth.

3.1. Definition and Symptoms

Some women could have just a couple of symptoms or a few of them. A genetic basis for catching postpartum depression is another theory. Women who have a mother, sister, or aunt who has had postpartum depression are at a greater risk for the condition. Many individuals believe that hormone fluctuations during pregnancy and after delivery may induce postpartum depression. However, evidence suggests that a complex network of physiological and behavioral causes, as well as the emotional aspects of delivery, have a significant effect. After birth, women's pressure and hormonal levels suddenly decrease. Women's moods may change as they adapt to having an infant and going through major lifestyle adjustments.

Postpartum depression (PPD) is a type of mood disorder connected with birth. The mood disorder is not just attributable to the dramatic hormonal modifications that occur before delivery and right after birth, but a variety of variables and possible causes. Postpartum depression is thus likely to occur from childbirth mishaps. Symptoms are mainly depressed mood, anxiety, and loss of joy that can hinder a woman's ability to take care of herself or her family. Symptoms may include being unable to connect with their baby, not reflecting thoughts about suicide, getting angry and annoyed, feeling powerless and not worth it, and more.

3.2. Risk Factors and Causes

Poor or lack of support system - It can be especially hard on women who are made to feel the primary caregiver in today's world of do everything by the neighbor who follows outdated "mom knows best." It's normal to only want the best for your baby, but different doesn't mean wrong. Each mother, and each child, are unique, and Mother Nature will usually let you know when something is horribly wrong. Unrealistic expectations of motherhood or the father not being able to provide emotional support - you're a dad. Not taking care of yourself - When you're busy these days, with doctor's appointments, baby showers, breastfeeding classes, buying diapers, grew supply plus learning to cloth diaper and seriously? You thought that breastfeeding might be the easy way out and you'd try everything else first...wow! The last thing you are going to think of - though it is probably the most important part - is YOURSELF.

Stressful events - During the early weeks and often the advance of the final trimester, many women are hit with a huge dose of stress. Whether it be family death, the death of a close family pet, house/homeschooling moving, a difficult separation, money problems, or even just dealing with family, stress can affect anyone during pregnancy. Your lack of good sleep might not only cause postpartum depression but may also lead to post-traumatic stress disorder after childbirth, especially if the stress is coupled with a traumatic birth experience.

History of anxiety or depression - Previous or ongoing struggles with depression or anxiety can significantly contribute to the likelihood of experiencing postpartum depression. Women who have experienced symptoms of depression prior to or during pregnancy are more likely to suffer from postpartum depression.

4. Key Similarities

Symptoms such as crying, anxiety, and moodiness are alike for both mothers with postpartum depression and those with the baby blues. Whether mothers have the baby blues or postpartum depression, in most scenarios, they will withdraw from things like yardwork, household chores, and recreation. They may also lose joy and interest in simple activities. Furthermore, some mothers struggle with issues when concentrating and making decisions. The stigma behind postpartum depression is also the same as the stigma that comes with the baby blues. For new moms, postpartum depression is a subject that nobody talks about, suggesting that it is a taboo or non-existent problem.

Although the baby blues and postpartum depression are two distinct occurrences, they have several fundamental similarities. Most notably, both focus on the parent that has just had the baby. These two feelings of depression can overlap; someone having postpartum depression may also be experiencing the baby blues, or vice versa. Both conditions can arise from hormonal changes. An ovulation-inducing hormone called estradiol is at its highest levels after birth, and a lactation-induced hormone called progesterone is at its lowest. Another hormone, called prolactin, which is responsible for the production of milk, also decreases. In both instances, adrenaline levels are affected, which can induce anxiety. Because of hormone distribution, premenopausal women are more prone to mood changes. These similarities between the baby blues and postpartum depression suggest a vast grey area between them, which is neither one nor the other.

Key Similarities

5. Key Differences

Thirdly, while the depressed new mother suffering from the baby blues will quite often feel a peak and trough of emotional symptoms within the span of a day, someone suffering from postpartum depression could experience this pattern once or twice a day. It is far more likely that the symptoms of postpartum depression will carry on throughout the day without ever lifting. Likewise, someone with postpartum depression will often experience symptoms ranging from really bad to bedside themselves in a matter of hours, or vice versa.

Another criterion for postpartum depression that is not seen in the baby blues is other feelings of frustration, hopelessness, and dejection. Furthermore, these symptoms will usually interfere with the several daily activities of the recovering mother. Postpartum depression differs from baby blues symptoms, such as extreme fatigue and feelings of mild guilt, as well as setting unrealistic goals for herself and then being dissatisfied. Postpartum depression can have symptoms severe enough to interfere with normal activities.

A major criterion just recently mentioned is the duration of the symptoms. In order to be classified as having postpartum depression, the patient will display signs at least 2 weeks after delivery. While the baby blues will disappear roughly after a week, someone dealing with true postpartum depression is functioning with unrelenting and unremitting symptoms.

6. Impact on Mothers and Families

Unlike the baby blues, for which social support and shared understanding can be helpful, with PPD sympathetic support from others, and from professionals is a must. Medication and/or counseling are the recommended treatment. Postpartum depression and the baby blues can cause mothers countless discomfort. The emotional, psychological, social, and economic cost of these conditions, however, needs to be thought about, felt, measured, and appreciated as a national public health problem, and not just an individual issue for the mother. Postpartum depression is real. It is serious. It is treatable. It has been widely researched and is well-understood in many ways.

Postpartum depression (PPD) is a serious mental illness that usually affects mothers within days of her baby's birth but can develop any time in the weeks or months after the baby is born. Depressed mothers' babies are less likely to thrive. They may eat less and have more sleep problems. The mother-infant bond can be affected as well, which can cause issues in school, in social relationships, and with overall health that can persist into childhood and the teenage years. The mother may feel that she wants to hurt her baby or that she regrets being a mother and may feel suicidal.

The baby blues imitate or give way to other mental illnesses such as postpartum depression or postpartum psychosis. Postpartum psychosis is much less common and can cause delusions, hallucinations, agitation, moods of extreme energy, depression, anxiety, and strange behavior as early as the first few days after birth. Symptoms are usually severe and last for a short time if they are treated appropriately. But if a woman develops these severe symptoms, it is of the utmost importance to get help right away.

7. Diagnosis and Screening

The Edinburgh Postnatal Depression Scale (EPDS) is one of the most widely-used postpartum depression screening instruments in practice today. Developed in 1987, the EPDS is a 10-item self-report scale designed as a screening instrument for depression in the perinatal and postnatal period. This 10-item questionnaire is both reliable and valid, making it easy to use and score by healthcare professionals. The purpose of the EPDS is to identify perinatal mood concerns present in a peripartum and postpartum patient. This scale can also be administered periodically throughout the postpartum period to reassess a patient when in doubt about her mental wellness. Early identification and early intervention are essential.

Diagnosing the baby blues can be difficult, as no lab tests are designed specifically for the baby blues. However, by diagnosing via the process of elimination, the doctor will rule out postpartum depression as well as postpartum psychosis, at which point the diagnosis of baby blues will be made with the understanding that no further treatment is necessary, as the baby blues does not usually require medical intervention. To properly assess whether a woman is suffering from baby blues or from postpartum depression, it is vital that her healthcare provider screens for peripartum and postpartum mood disorders throughout the antenatal and postnatal period. Without detection and early intervention, postpartum depression is likely to ensue. Unfortunately, only 17% of antenatal and

8% of postpartum women are currently being screened for perinatal mood disorders in most obstetrical/gynecological settings.

8. Treatment and Interventions

Many people develop the baby blues, yet some may need treatment to face it. Sometimes a person's lifestyle or a simple personality trait causes normal feelings to become more intense. Postpartum depression is generally more severe, and treatment has to be taken very seriously as it can lead to death. Medications tend to have side effects and may cause birth defects, and they may be passed through breastfeeding, so medications are usually a tough choice for a new mom. For example, art therapy is also used in dysthymia and major depressive disorder. People with peripartum onset major depression or loss of a baby may also attend support groups that are designed to help, but more research is needed to determine the impact of such interaction.

Medical professionals tend to treat the baby blues with treatment that addresses the physical changes during pregnancy and childbirth, as well as the physical changes to moods and hormones. As for postpartum depression, there are many approaches possible that may be taken to help a patient through it. Some patients may try therapy to get at the root of their feelings and to talk through their concerns. There are also many antidepressant medications and other medications for the anxiety and panic that some people may suffer from. Doctors generally also take a holistic approach, having some patients work with experts to address nutrition, sleep, and stress. A popular topic that is still being studied is the benefits of working with an art therapist and expressing oneself to overcome postpartum depression.

9. Support and Resources

For general information on common perinatal mood disorders (including postpartum depression, up and down mood, and anxiety), call the PSI Warmline at 1-800-944-4773 (4PPD). This number will connect you with someone who has received specialized training on perinatal mood disorders and mood disorders support. Don't be afraid to call. The sooner you talk to someone, the quicker you're likely to get the proper diagnosis and an individualized treatment plan put in place. And the more quickly your symptoms are addressed, the better you can feel.

Having a strong support network to help you through this challenging time is critical to your recovery, according to the Centers for Disease Control. If you're feeling down, seek help. Contact your doctor, or reach out to a family member, friend, or postpartum support group. They can help you find the resources you need and offer support as you go through the treatment process. The knowledge that you're not alone can provide a significant emotional boost and take some of the sting out of what you're going through. Local postpartum support groups may have referrals and recommendations for professionals in and around your area. Postpartum Support International offers evidence-based information on perinatal mood and anxiety disorders, provides free support, and has mailing lists for healthcare providers, mood disorders support groups, and anxiety support.

If you're experiencing the tedium, mixed emotions, fatigue, and sense of isolation that can occur post-birth, know that you're not alone, and that what you're experiencing, be it the baby blues or postpartum depression, is a medical condition that has effective treatment options available to you.

10. Cultural and Societal Perspectives

Maternal mental instability has resulted in large numbers of children worldwide becoming unintentional collateral damage of the Cold War, and in a growing number of cases in antenatal or postpartum infanticide in the 21st century. In the early WRA case reports, recommended advice included increasing the socioeconomic status of unwanted out of wedlock mothers and wives, usually at the cost of the biological father. Accurate reporting of WRA statistics can also be obscured by the cultural need of some societies to support the mother-and-infant dyad at all costs. Concealment of maternal psychological distress and abnormal parenting has been demonstrated in India and Pakistan to overcome any cultural, societal, or family concerns about the mental health of some antenatal, postpartum, and other caregivers of children that deviate from the rigorous blueprint of expectant and societal parenting.

In general, postpartum health is defined by monitoring the physical, psychological, and social wellbeing of the mother and baby. However, relatively little is known or discussed about the impact of prenatal, antenatal, and postpartum negative emotional wellbeing (e.g., in low-income countries) on motherhood. In most developed societies, however, it is expected that postpartum women will be affected by tearfulness or dysphoria after childbirth. Indeed, the 'Baby Blues' is a Western psychiatric disorder with symptoms of mild, unpleasant mood disturbance following childbirth, and the cultural context predicts temporary feelings of anxiety, tiredness, and reduced concentration in the first 2 days after giving birth. The UN's 1955 Geneva Convention outlawed the effect of warfare on mothers and babies during the childbearing year. Implicitly, this definition implies that the younger and older childbearing cohorts will or should be vocal and immune from the wars of activism that may induce temporary depressive feelings following childbirth.

11. Research and Future Directions

Postpartum depression is associated with many different physiological, environmental, social, and psychological characteristics. In 2019, we have already seen more research directly involving the baby blues, which is a significant step forward in increasing our knowledge and being able to help the women who develop this adjustment disorder. Moving forward, these findings need to be further validated as the research is in its absolute infancy and associated with relatively small sample sizes and some methodological limitations. In particular, because recent work has reported results from Samoa, which is typically used to suggest that the baby blues is not a severe phenomenon and is resolved within the early postpartum period, it is important to reassess the time course of this condition and the statistical methodology employed. A meta-analysis and review of the literature may also be able to shed some light on potential new directions for research into the baby blues. Other work will be the start of initial examination of supportive interventions for women experiencing the baby blues in comparison to an active psychological placebo. JBM-TD research in the area of baby blues is a fast-moving area, and I am sure it won't be long until we see more interesting new papers that can be discussed in 2020.

Research efforts have focused primarily on the physiological and related emotional processes. While some researchers have focused on the differences in biomarker expression between women with and without the baby blues, typically those without reducers are in the minority and would not be useful to corroborate that the baby blues are a normal response to having a baby. Other key differences that have been suggested as factors contributing towards the development of the baby blues in different women include complications at birth, the onset of sleep disturbances, and less social/familial support.

12. Conclusion

When the fourth trimester is over and a mother is still
feeling the same, she should never hesitate to reach out.
Whether or not the feelings were just rolling over into the
more pathological depression, or if they have been there all
along, it does not matter. The point is that help will still be
received. More frequently, women go untreated because of
being scared about the opinion of others. Prioritizing the
most vulnerable individual over the false judgment of
others is crucial when there are bigger fish to fry. It is okay
and healthy to seek help if it is what is best for you and
your family. Ensuring a woman knows that she is not alone
and that there are others who have gone through or are
going through the same thoughts and postpartum
symptoms is the most important aspect. This paper truly
gets down to the nitty and gritty of it all as mothers need it.

The baby blues can be very close to postpartum
depression, but they can also be very far apart. It is
important that new mothers know that these feelings are
much more common than one may think. The heart-
wrenching feelings of not being a good enough mother are
enough to scare anyone into thinking that they are alone.
Knowing that it is more than normal to be feeling these
symptoms might alleviate the tension women are putting
on themselves.

Understanding and Addressing Postpartum Depression

1. Introduction to Postpartum Depression

Postpartum depression (PPD) is a debilitating and far-reaching disorder affecting many women in the wake of the landmark event of the birth of a child. The hormonal changes regulating pregnancy do seem to influence the possibility of developing the disorder. No known determinant of postpartum depression, genetic or otherwise, has been located to date. Rather than physically causing the disorder, the genetic makeup predisposes one to develop depression as a negative reaction to the stressful events associated with postpartum experiences. The cut-off date of up to 3 months postpartum for postpartum depression may have initially been thought to permanently end the disease and the mother's debilitating feelings of hopelessness for good, but 10 years has shown that this is a fallacy.

Introduction: Postpartum depression is a common and disabling disorder that often goes undiscovered and untreated. Although psychosocial and hormonal changes related to the birth of a child play a role in the development of the disorder, the exact etiology of postpartum depression has yet to be identified. Known to be a significant risk factor for major depression in women, postpartum depression should be taken very seriously. This paper will analyze the causes and genetic factors of postpartum depression, along with the cultural blame of the mother by examining different societies, social standards, and healthcare beliefs. We will also discuss the current outdated method of screening for postpartum depression and appropriate up-to-date treatment.

2. Signs and Symptoms

Because levels of estrogen and progesterone quickly drop after childbirth, a new mother is especially likely to experience overlapping signs and symptoms of postpartum depression and mood swings. However, as time passes, if the depression is not successfully treated, symptoms featured may not be limited to mood problems, a lack of energy, and frequent sleep disturbances. Women who have not experienced improvements in their condition in the 1 to 4 months after giving birth may go on to experience significant weight loss when not dieting or unexpected weight gain or a decrease or increase in appetite. They may feel much less sexually interested in sex than in the past, or else that it is difficult or impossible to reach orgasm. They may sleep excessively or struggle to get the rest they need, may often be fidgety or else spend several hours immobile, tired, or physically slowed down.

First and foremost, persistent and severe feelings of sadness, hopelessness, anxiety, emptiness, anger, or irritability are hallmarks of postpartum depression. Feelings of excessive or unwarranted fear, decreased interest or pleasure in activities one used to enjoy, such as time with loved ones or caring for one's baby, are common, as is the expectation that nothing will ever get better. Changes in appetite and/or weight, drinking more or less, being unable to sleep or sleeping too much, and physical symptoms that do not have a clear cause, such as stomachaches and headaches, are also frequently experienced. A woman with postpartum depression is likely to struggle with thinking and concentrating and with making decisions, and she may have restless or slowed-down movements.

2.1. Baby Blues vs. Postpartum Depression

In terms of depression alone, the rates of postpartum depression are lower than antenatal depression, with only 13% of women being diagnosed with major depression after childbirth. Postpartum depression can show up any time in the first year after childbirth and the longest duration of decades. It can also range from mild to life-threatening, with serviced women being referred to the associated healthcare services. It is important to be cautious when talking about postpartum depression, as abnormalities in cognitive, affective, and reward systems make it radically different from other forms of depression. Additionally, it is trenchant to acknowledge that parents or primary carers with same-sex partners and transgender individuals can also experience postpartum depression, although this conversation lies beyond the scope of this article.

Pregnancy, childbirth, or postpartum mental health remain understated conversations in most societies, nonetheless impacting the emotional and mental life of parents. Here, we will address just one facet of postpartum mental health - postpartum depression - in detail. However, it is important to first distinguish between the often experienced 'baby blues' and postpartum depression. Baby blues is a period characterized by mood swings, mild euphoria, irritability, and anxiety that comes 3 - 5 days after childbirth and generally subsides within a week or ten days. On the other hand, postpartum depression is conditions such as anxiety disorder, post-traumatic stress disorder, phobia, panic disorder.

3. Risk Factors

Several triggers for the depression have been identified besides the hormonal changes that follow birth. Others think that women who are prone to postpartum depression may have a history of depression or similar illnesses, had the illness in a previous pregnancy, have family members with mood disturbances, are experiencing increased stress caused by the demands of the baby, or feel fatigued. Women of all ages can develop postpartum depression, but teenage mothers seem to be at greater risk. Some studies have shown that women who are not married, live alone, have financial problems, or lack social support are at a higher risk for postpartum depression. The birth of a child has an impact on any family, and fathers are just as likely as a mother to suffer from postpartum depression. The main risk factors for depression in men are having a history of depression, experiencing anger or emotional upset during the pregnancy, or feeling stressed or anxious. Other possible causes of depression may include the following: inadequacy or poor preparation to take on parental responsibilities, feelings of helplessness, and concern about the ability to care for and support his family, fear of being overshadowed by the baby, or discomfort with changes in his partner's sexual activity or attractiveness. Stressful home events, financial problems, or other changes related to a new baby can also contribute to a father's depression.

The arrival of a newborn is typically a joyful time for the whole family, but new mothers may not feel like celebrating if they have postpartum depression. More than just feeling irritable and weepy, the condition is a type of depression that presents with feelings of sadness, worthlessness, and withdrawal from one's family.

4. Impact on Parent and Child

The potential effects of postpartum depression on the child are also widespread. Children of parents with postpartum depression have been found to score lower on cognitive development and verbal ability compared to children of healthy parents, and may have temperamental or behavioral differences. One study which examined maternal depressive symptoms found that such symptoms are inversely associated with the child's IQ at age 3, and such symptoms are also associated with the child's IQ later in life. It is worth noting, however, that the child's father may be able to mediate this effect by providing a greater support system. Another study found that mothers diagnosed with postpartum depression have lower parenting self-efficacy and that this results in more often bringing the child to the doctor even when the child is not sick.

The potential effects of postpartum depression on the parent are vast. For many individuals struggling with postpartum depression, the postpartum period is a time of increased anxiety, self-doubt, and uncertainty. Furthermore, postpartum depression is a significant predictor of depression in both the short-term and the long-term, and one study found that mothers with postpartum depression are at a higher risk of suicide than the general population. Postpartum depression may also generate shame in the parent, exacerbating the effects of the already stigmatized disorder. For many parents, postpartum depression can result in difficulty emotionally connecting to the child, frustration, and feeling unable to adequately care for the child. For those who experience bipolar depression, those symptoms can be significantly pronounced.

5. Diagnosis and Screening

Postpartum depression is best captured in its earliest stages. It is recommended by a number of organizations, including the American Academy of Pediatrics, that all mothers be screened in their infant's birth hospital by the pediatric services. A number of specific screeners exist for postpartum depression, but some of the most popular ones with good psychometric properties include the Edinburgh Postpartum Depression Scale (EPDS), the Patient Health Questionnaire (PHQ-9), and the Postpartum Depression Screening Scale (PDSS). It is more common than not for a healthcare provider to inquire with the new mother about symptoms since childbirth, sleep problems, or other possible indicators of postpartum depression without using a specific measure at the very minimum for a complete review. Postpartum depression is assessed on a three-tiered scale within the journey of childbirth and varies in duration and is specified in the Diagnostic and Statistical Manual of Mental Disorders (DSM-5) as Major Depressive Disorder, with peripartum onset. At its height, postpartum depression has a high incidence of anxiety, panic, and intrusive thoughts and hallucinations involving harm to the baby, called "postpartum anxieties" or "postpartum OCD" if a compulsive behavior is used to manage the intrusive thought. To go over the diagnosis and screening methods would take an article of its own, but it is important for the reader to find the information for themselves if needed with the other resources at the end of this paper.

Postpartum depression is a complex mix of physical, emotional, and behavioral changes that interfere with a woman's ability to function and impacts not only her life but her child's life and subsequently the family unit as well. It is primarily a diagnosis associated with women who have given birth in the past 12 months, but it can develop before childbirth, be found in non-birth parents, and if not addressed effectively, can persist much longer. Incidence rates vary, but most research is clear in showing that about 15% of all new mothers and at least 10% of new fathers will fulfill criteria for postpartum depression at some point. Long-term consequences of the condition include suboptimal parent-infant bonding, child emotional and behavioral problems, and suppression of the child's immune system, to name a few. There is valuable help in various locations for the mother to address her symptoms, but first, the condition must be captured.

6. Treatment Options

Given the complex nature of postpartum depression, a combination of strategies and interventions is often required. Therapy can aim to increase helpful activity and reduce seclusive, avoidant, or indulgent behavior. Strategies can include pacing activities, organizing childcare, increasing structured practical demands, problem solving and cognitive skills training (reasoning, internal dialogue, and reappraisal). This can also be carried out in a group context, which can include other new mothers. To have a beneficial effect, a group would need to offer mutual support and the facilitator would need to create a situation where help-giving is regarded as an indication of strength rather than an admission of failure. A therapist training yoga therapy initially will need the same level of training required of Interpersonal Therapists.

There are a number of treatment options available for postpartum depression. Given the fluctuating time frame of hormonal changes, a treatment addressing neurobiological contributors and context of transition to motherhood may be particularly beneficial. Objectives of treatment intervention can include addressing the neurobiological contributors, addressing the accompanying maladaptive depressive cognitions and behavior, creating space for developing helpful family dynamics and practical strategies, and supporting the transition to motherhood. This can follow dose escalation and/or change to a medication from a different class, if required. Around 20%

to 30% of women will need ECT or other advanced treatments and a significant proportion will need to switch to a different medication class before an improvement is seen. Thus, treatment can take time to act and the family, practical, and psychological issues created by the symptoms will need to be managed.

Cognitive Therapy. Cognitive-behavioral therapy is based on a very simple idea: the way we think about things affects how we feel emotionally. Therefore, if we can change our thinking who are negative or unrealistic to thinking that are more positive, hopeful, and realistic, we can make ourselves feel better. Cognitive-behavioral therapists use a number of techniques to help change negative thinking patterns about the self, the world, and the future. The first step is to identify the kinds of situations, events, people, places, or things that seem to cause depressed feelings. The second step is to become aware of what sorts of negative thoughts might be "popping into" your mind when you encounter these "triggers." In many cases, these negative thoughts may be so habitual that you are not even consciously aware of them. The final step is to learn how these thoughts are related to your mood.

Treatment for postpartum depression can be divided into several different types, one of which is therapy or counseling. Postpartum women who were depressed during pregnancy are those who have been found to benefit the most from these types of treatments from direct research. Although therapy and counseling can be expensive or difficult to obtain, they can be very helpful in reducing symptoms of postpartum depression. Therapy and counseling can also help women who are unable to take medication due to breastfeeding or other medical conditions. Psychological therapy is also known as "talk therapy," referring to treatments that involve talking to a psychologist or therapist about your thoughts, feelings, and behaviors. Specific forms of psychological therapy that are effective in treating postpartum depression include cognitive-behavioral therapy (CBT) and interpersonal therapy (IPT), which are described in more detail below.

6.2. Medication

- Antidepressants: Several studies have concluded that antidepressants can be effective for the treatment of postpartum depression. Selective serotonin reuptake inhibitors (SSRIs) are the most researched in relation to this. It has been noted that SSRI breastmilk levels, and therefore infant exposure, can range from 8-70% of maternal serum levels. For this reason, and due to severe reactions seen in up to 15% of exposed newborns, we do not prescribe Paxil (paroxetine) to mothers who are breastfeeding. We also recommend against Zoloft (sertraline) due to observed short half-life, breastmilk levels averaging 27-38% of maternal serum levels and association with infant reactions. Similar half-lives are seen with Effexor (venlafaxine) meaning it, and its metabolite, can concentrate in breastmilk and may cause severe reactions in the nursing infant. Lexapro (escitalopram) is probably the safest for breastfeeding as it has a lower excretion rate compared to other antidepressants. There have been no documented reports of accumulation in breastmilk, infant toxicity, or vanishing seizures, and very few detectable reactions in nursing infants. While there are a variety of antidepressant medications, these are some of the most common ones. A family physician will be best able to determine which is best for an individual based on a variety of factors.

Pharmacological Interventions

Postpartum depression is often severe and can significantly impact a mother's ability to care for their infant. Considering that, it is not unreasonable to consider medication, especially if depression symptoms come on abruptly or are recurrent. That being said, many mothers may be hesitant about taking anything while breastfeeding. Several things should be considered prior to initiating a medication.

7. Support Systems and Resources

Many factors contribute. An aggressive reproductive system that allows for a shorter postpartum period, rather than infirms you to the point where the only option for moving forward is support; for many, a veritable lack of support systems or resources; accentuated feelings of guilt, sadness, anger, or anxiety over postpartum birth complications, stillbirths, cesarean sections, or inability to conceive; and environmental factors like mothers who depend on welfare. Any of the following can make a change in the health levels of the mother and the infant. Any of the following can increase the likelihood of postpartum depression by 50% if a woman scores 12 or higher with a postpartum depression quiz. Therefore, women must ask for help.

Claiming neither a simple cure nor a direct cause, postpartum depression is still very difficult both as a patient and as a family member. "Sometimes, to call it only a problem with the thyroid is not the whole truth. To say it's only a psychological issue isn't entirely true either. Sometimes it's because you're dead tired and not sleeping and sometimes it's because you don't have a partner, or you are under so much stress from worrying about this or that," said Sally Barraj. Around 8% of women are impacted by postpartum depression.

8. Prevention Strategies

A multitude of interventions and strategies have been proposed, including universal screening, selective or risk-based screening (i.e., screening specifically for certain clinical or demographic factors), treatment of symptomatic women, and prevention programs aimed at reducing the occurrence of depressive symptoms in women who are subthreshold for a clinical diagnosis of depression. Given the predominance of prenatal symptoms and subthreshold depression in the epidemiologic surveys cited above, prevention strategies likely play a key role in lowering the occurrence of postpartum depression (PPD). In the remainder of this review, we provide an overview of the literature on proposed prevention strategies for the development of PPD.

As penalties of prenatal exposure to anxiety/depressive states arise almost as predominant as postpartum depression (PPD), and as late pregnancy and the first postpartum components are associated with neurodevelopmental effects, preventive approaches are warranted. Psychological treatments for subclinical states are preventively effective and likely to be cost-effective. While preventive programs are likely to be acceptable to pregnant women and society, maternal health care workers do not have the resources to guarantee their implementation or to diagnose mother and child. Information interventions based on psychoeducation, self-care or lifestyle change, universal screening, and treatment indicate indicated interventions could be part of optimal preventive care. Maternity care can become more involved in preventive maternal mental health care as vaccine prevention becomes available alongside treatment strategies. The prevention of prenatal depression is currently limited by the absence of studies conducted to high methodological and reporting standards. It is likely that psychological treatments for subclinical states are preventively effective and cost-effective. More research is needed on the notification and treatment of services because they could be both public health and women-friendly. The major epidemiological and neurobiological 'windows' starting during pregnancy makes preventive efforts urgently needed.

9. Cultural and Societal Perspectives

Fear was commonly expressed that women with PPD could be seen as mad and would have no role in society. In general, women were less concerned about the stigma of being mentally ill as long as they were alive and able to take care of their home, children, and husband. Thus, community, interpersonal, and self-stigmatization risks play out differently depending on the local context, potential meaning of having a mental illness, and potentially risky behavior. When it comes to individual differences, there may be factors which enable people to serve as a stigma buffer. Receiving care or any type of help for PPD could both improve and diminish stigma as a woman may become understood as "needy" and hence more prone to stigma. In addition, the reliance on professional help could lead to the understanding that care has not been effective, increasing stigma further. Relevantly, community members appreciated that women in their village suffer and believe that public efforts should support them. Stigma was particularly high when they coupled her suffering with her husband's death, blamed her for her depression, threatened to hurt her, and avoided her in the community.

Even when trained using the most current official diagnostic criteria, psychiatrists from diverse cultural and societal backgrounds can differ in their diagnoses of PPD. A psychiatric perspective may lead to unfamiliarity in addressing the wide array of symptoms experienced among diverse client populations. Traditional birth attendant and community health worker perspectives have been identified as more inclusive of broader social and emotional struggles faced by women postpartum. For example, in Goa, India, social scientists have reported that depressed women are more likely to be diagnosed with "weakness (nejli)" by TBAs because hair fall, weakness, and irritability with other family members are the hallmark symptoms of PPD in Goa. Moreover, even recognizing and classifying women as mentally ill can be filtered through cultural perspectives on women, motherhood, and mental illness. Yet it is known that different cultural meanings influence individual women in unique ways.

10. Future Research Directions

As the primary pathway by which inflammation might reach the brain is through the maternal-fetal interface, we might see more work in the field of developmental neuroimmunology and the interaction of peripheral and central inflammation around the time of birth to understand how these events relate to subsequent maternal mental health. As the PPD field progresses, longitudinal imaging research looking at the multilevel prenatal and postnatal adaptive and maladaptive changes to help the brain reorganize during the prenatal and postnatal period to target interventions for PPD is sorely needed. Postpartum women experience rapidly changing hormonal landscapes that impact their mental health, including both dramatic changes in gonadal hormones as well as in the hypothalamus-pituitary-adrenal or stress hormones. Identifying when, across the perinatal period, women are experiencing maladaptive changes in their hormonal stress neuroendocrine systems that predict PPD is an area ripe for further research. Finally, time series data in the postpartum period to identify changing women's brain circuits and hormonal stress axis functioning are a novel avenue for PPD research.

Considering that 10-15% of women experience PPD, future research might explore novel directions in managing this substantial public health burden, including looking for additional risk biomarkers that would augment risk stratification or neurobiological targets for PPD prevention. For example, epigenetic research might reveal better predictive markers or suggest new preventive therapies for women at high risk for PPD. The microglia and immune system in PPD might be a ripe area for future research, particularly as it regards PPD interventions. As we have learned from clinical trials in major depressive disorder, targeting the immune system without sufficient grounds to assume it is a part of the pathomechanism of the condition, such as enrolling participants with high levels of systemic TNF or CRP, is not likely to bear fruit. Therefore, additional research focusing on PPD neuroimaging and peripheral biomarker stratified RCTs are sorely needed for the field to advance towards personalized medicine for PPD.